I0762825

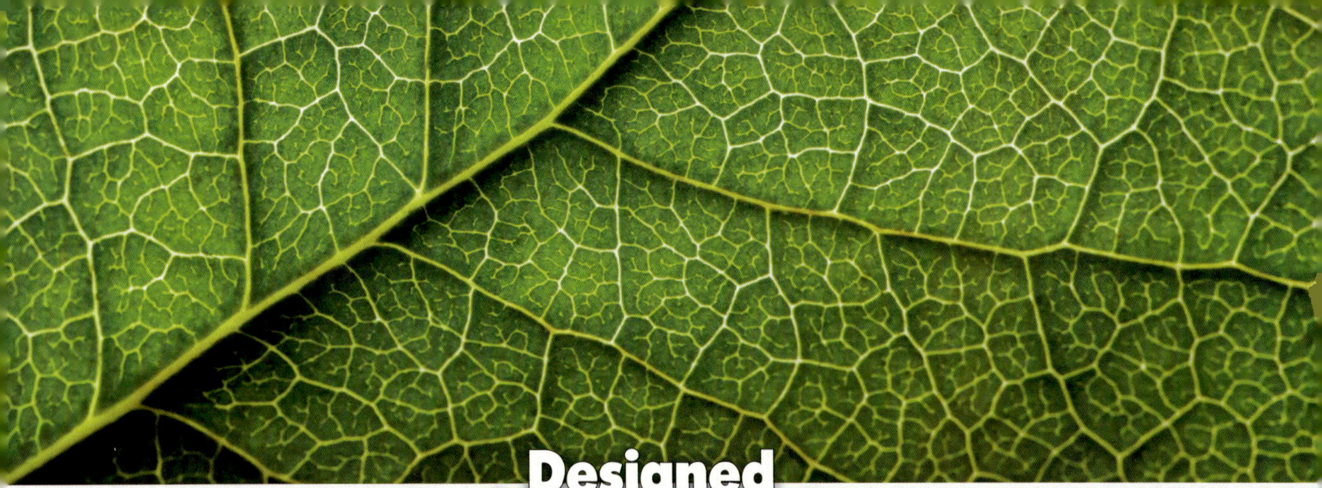

Designed by Nature

Medical Technology

Venessa Bellido Schwarz
and John Willis

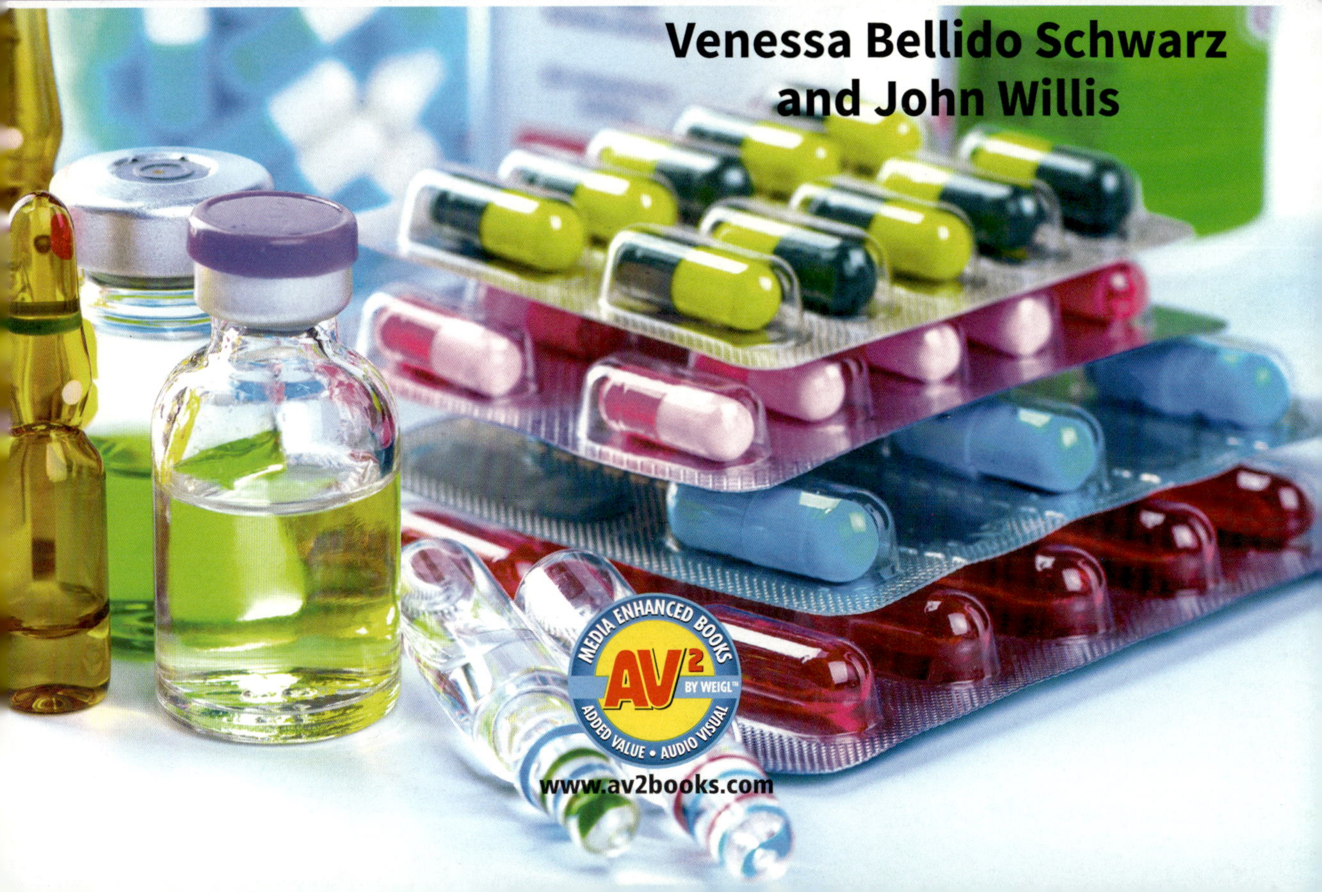

MEDIA ENHANCED BOOKS
AV2 BY WEIGL
ADDED VALUE • AUDIO VISUAL
www.av2books.com

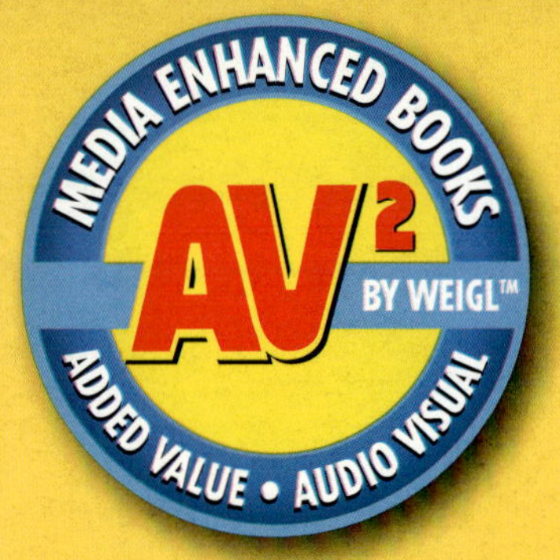

Go to www.av2books.com, and enter this book's unique code.

BOOK CODE

AVY75737

AV² by Weigl brings you media enhanced books that support active learning.

AV² provides enriched content that supplements and complements this book. Weigl's AV² books strive to create inspired learning and engage young minds in a total learning experience.

Your AV² Media Enhanced books come alive with...

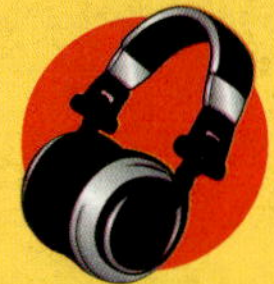

Audio
Listen to sections of the book read aloud.

Key Words
Study vocabulary, and complete a matching word activity.

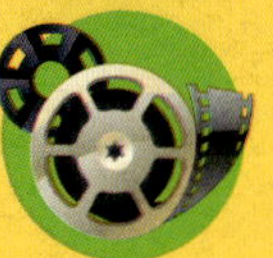

Video
Watch informative video clips.

Quizzes
Test your knowledge.

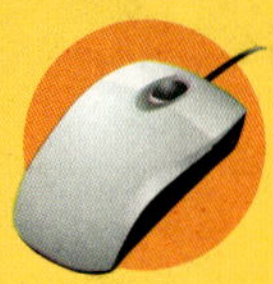

Embedded Weblinks
Gain additional information for research.

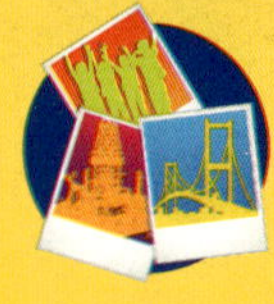

Slide Show
View images and captions, and prepare a presentation.

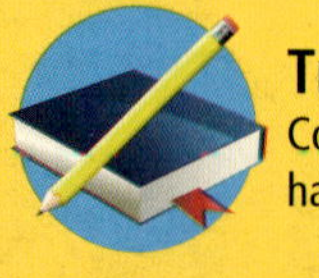

Try This!
Complete activities and hands-on experiments.

... and much, much more!

Published by AV² by Weigl
350 5th Avenue, 59th Floor
New York, NY 10118
Website: www.av2books.com

Library of Congress Cataloging-in-Publication Data
Names: Schwarz, Venessa Bellido, author. | Willis, John, author.
Title: Medical technology / Venessa Bellido Schwarz, John Willis.
Other titles: Medical technology inspired by nature
Description: New York, NY : AV2 by Weigl, [2019] | Series: Designed by nature | Audience: Grade 4 to 6. | Revision of: Medical technology inspired by nature. 2019. | Includes index.
Identifiers: LCCN 2018053543 (print) | LCCN 2018056483 (ebook) | ISBN 9781489697271 (Multi User Ebook) | ISBN 9781489697288 (Single User Ebook) | ISBN 9781489697257 (hardcover : alk. paper) | ISBN 9781489697264 (softcover : alk. paper)
Subjects: LCSH: Medical technology--Juvenile literature.
Classification: LCC R855.4 (ebook) | LCC R855.4 .S39 2019a (print) | DDC 610.285--dc23
LC record available at https://lccn.loc.gov/2018053543

Printed in the United States of America in Brainerd, Minnesota
1 2 3 4 5 6 7 8 9 0 22 21 20 19 18

122018
102318

Project Coordinator: John Willis   Designer: Ana María Vidal

Every reasonable effort has been made to trace ownership and to obtain permission to reprint copyright material. The publishers would be pleased to have any errors or omissions brought to their attention so that they may be corrected in subsequent printings.

Weigl acknowledges Alamy, Getty Images, iStock, Shutterstock, and Wikimedia as its primary image suppliers for this title.

First published by North Star Editions in 2019

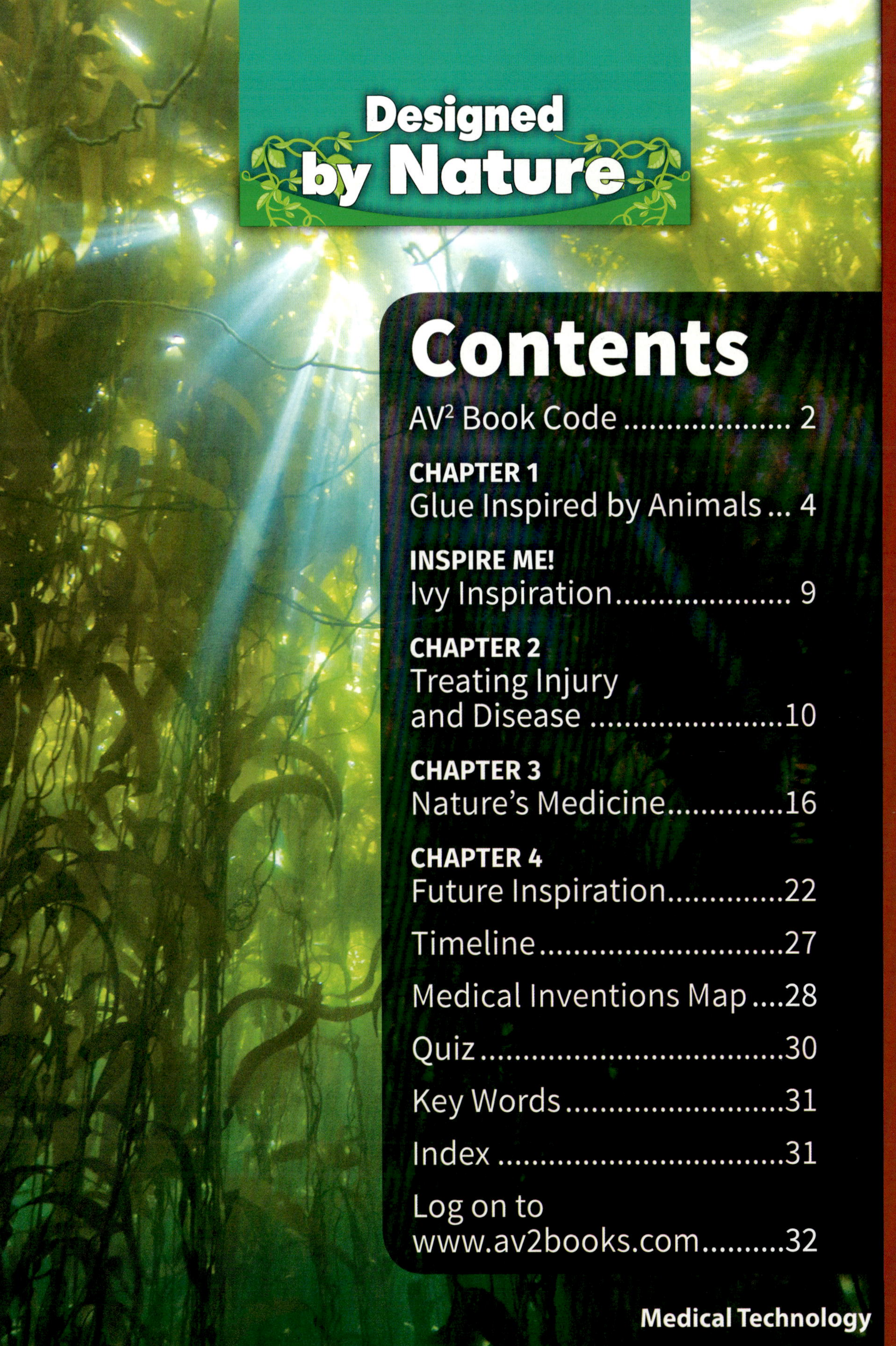

Contents

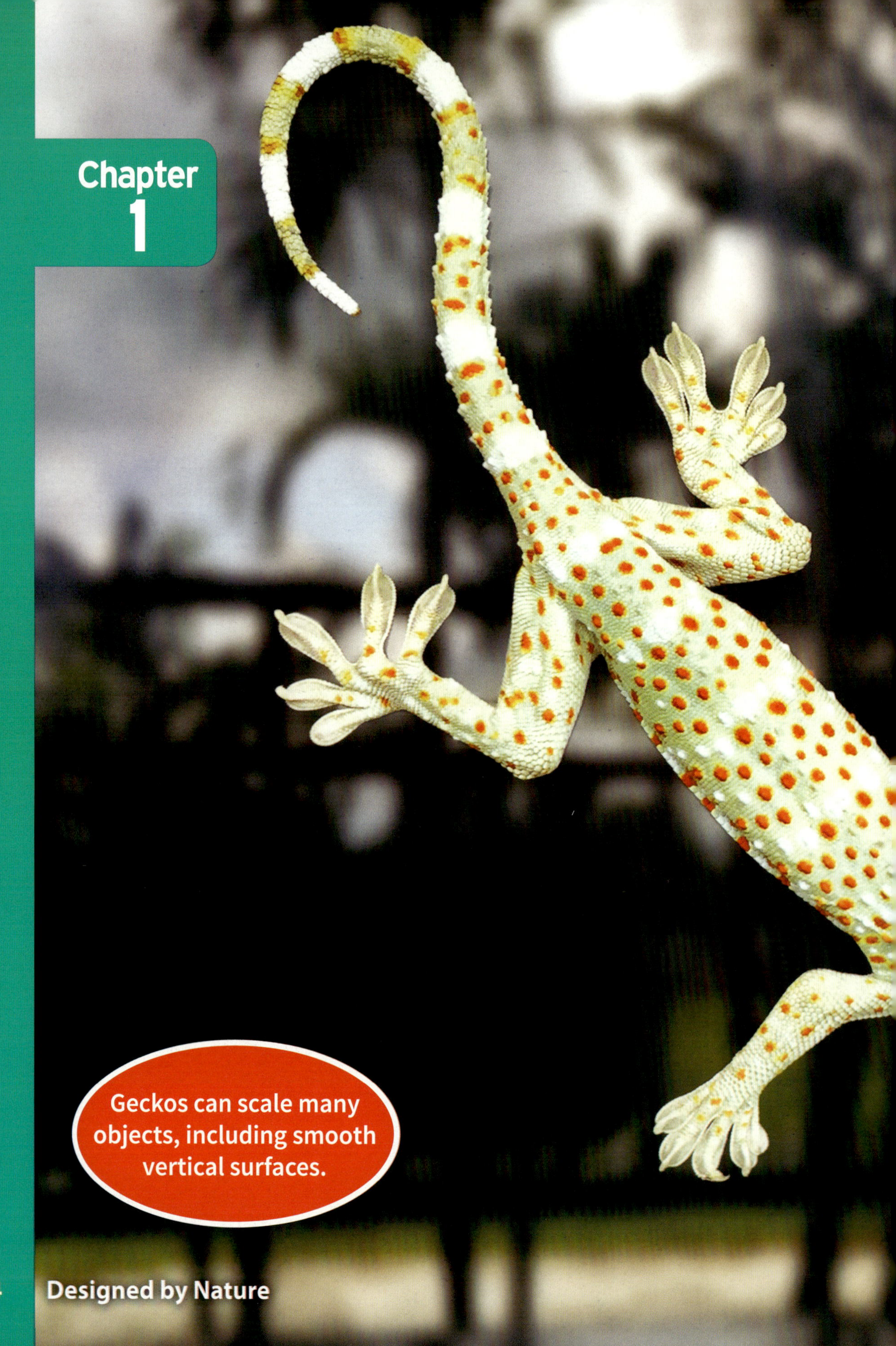

Chapter 1

Geckos can scale many objects, including smooth vertical surfaces.

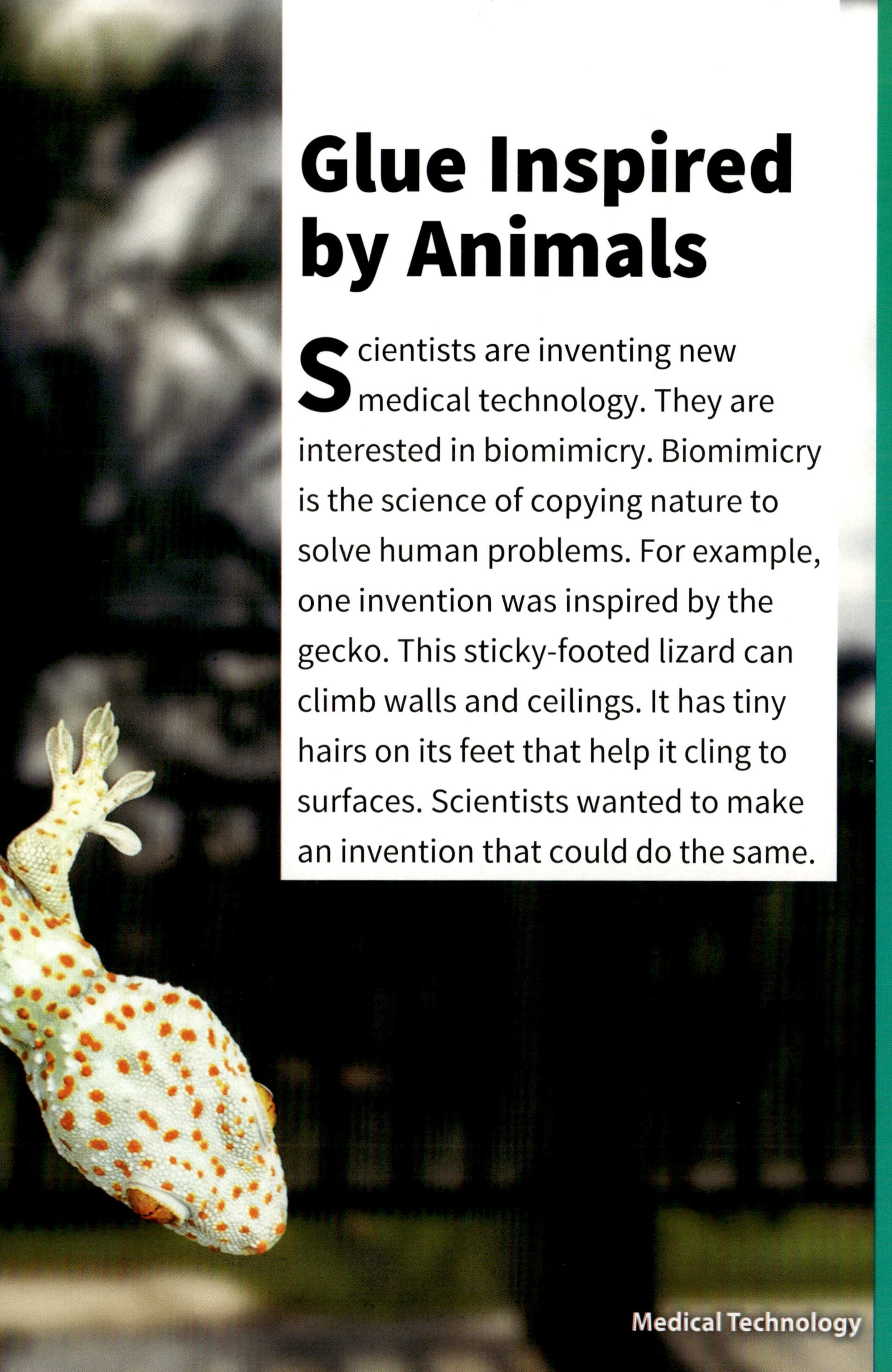

Glue Inspired by Animals

Scientists are inventing new medical technology. They are interested in biomimicry. Biomimicry is the science of copying nature to solve human problems. For example, one invention was inspired by the gecko. This sticky-footed lizard can climb walls and ceilings. It has tiny hairs on its feet that help it cling to surfaces. Scientists wanted to make an invention that could do the same.

Life-Changing Tape

Doctors have used gecko-inspired tapes since 2001. But the "gecko" tape invented in 2008 is different. As the tape breaks down, it puts medicine into the patient's body. It also causes less swelling than other tapes. When it is used on the skin, the tape comes off with ease. But when it is used inside the body, it dissolves into the bloodstream.

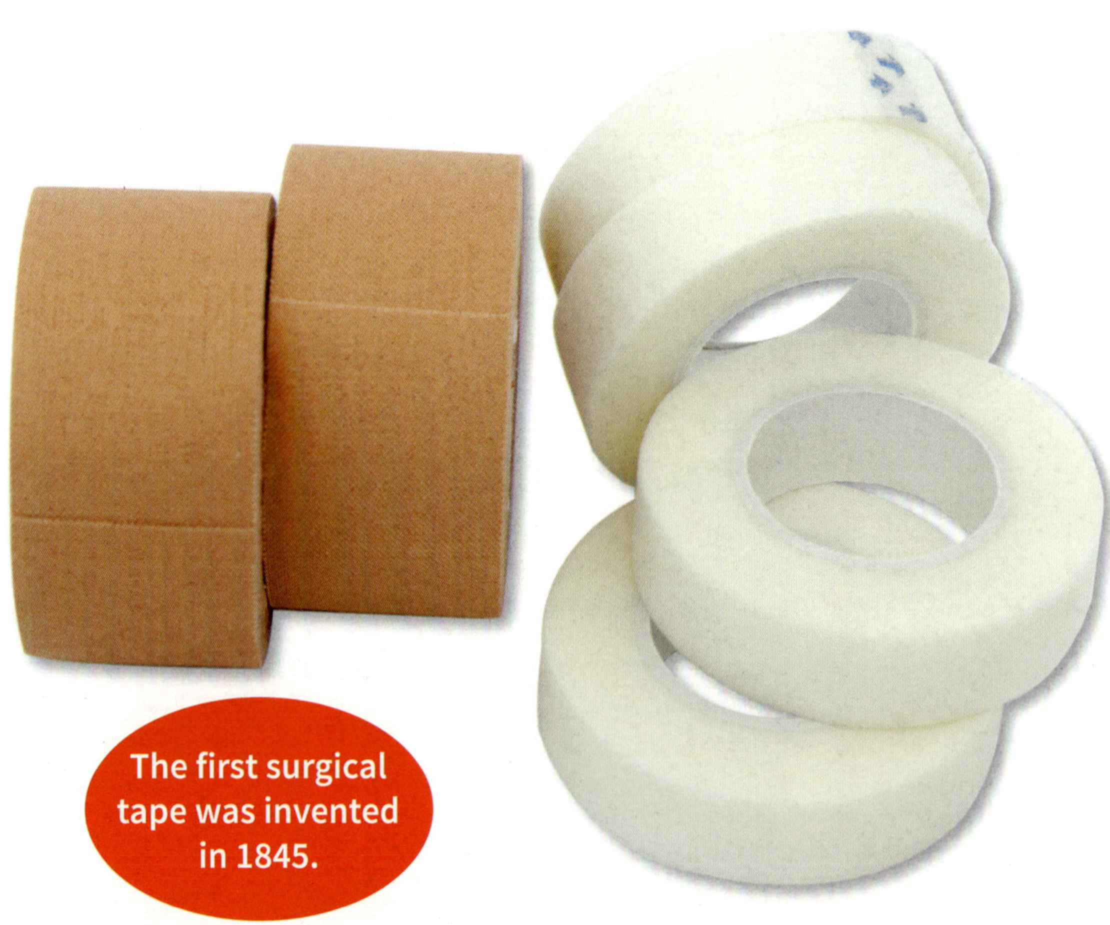

The first surgical tape was invented in 1845.

In 2008, one scientist invented a new type of surgical tape. The tape's surface is similar to a gecko's feet. The tape can help people who are injured. It bonds patients' wounds. The tape holds the wounds together so they can heal. Afterward, the tape comes off with ease.

One year later, the creator of the tape received a letter from a doctor at Boston Children's Hospital. The doctor worked with patients who had heart defects. He was struggling to seal holes in his patients' hearts. He needed glue stronger than the "gecko" tape.

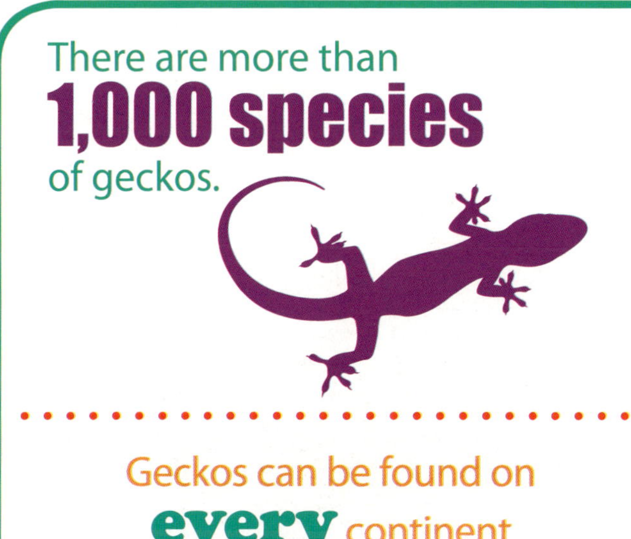

The largest geckos grow up to **14 inches** (35 centimeters) long.

Geckos can be found on **every** continent **except** for Antarctica.

Inventing this type of glue would be a challenge. The human heart is soaked with blood. It also moves forcefully as it pumps. But the scientist who received the letter was determined. Before long, he learned about the sandcastle worm.

This worm creates a sticky substance. The worm uses the substance to glue sand and seashells together underwater. The scientist and his team came up with an idea from it. They created a glue that repels water. The glue would soak into the heart and create a waterproof seal.

In 2016, four hospitals in France tested the glue. They tried to seal holes in the hearts of 36 patients. The glue worked well on the patients' beating hearts. The scientists' new invention was a success.

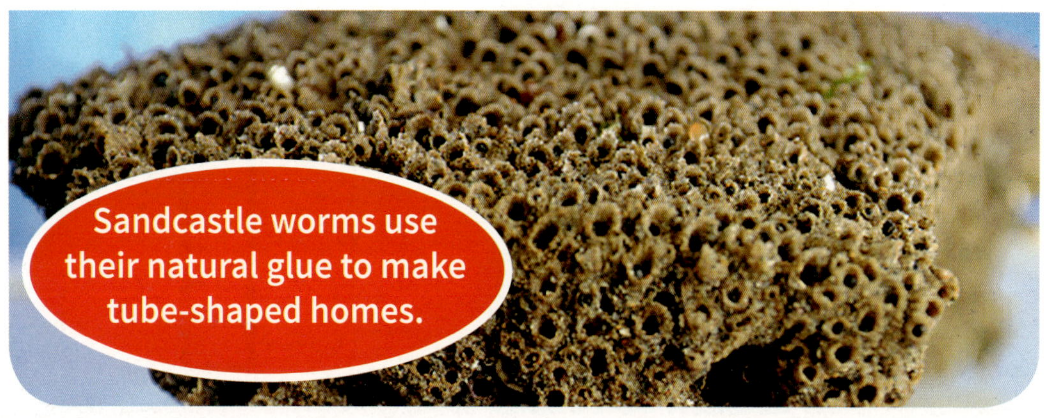

Sandcastle worms use their natural glue to make tube-shaped homes.

Inspire Me!

Ivy Inspiration

Ivy plants stick to the sides of buildings. The plants' roots dig into tiny cracks in the wall. Then they release a glue-like substance. The glue helps the plant hold on to the wall. As the ivy grows, it spreads in different directions.

The surgical glue inspired by the sandcastle worm works similarly. The glue seeps into the tiny cracks of an organ. Then it spreads in different directions. However, scientists struggled to hold the glue in place.

To fix the problem, the scientists invented a device that looks like a pen. The pen lets off a ray of light. This light makes the glue stay in place. The process takes less than five seconds.

Ivy roots change shape to fit the wall the plant is growing on.

Chapter 2

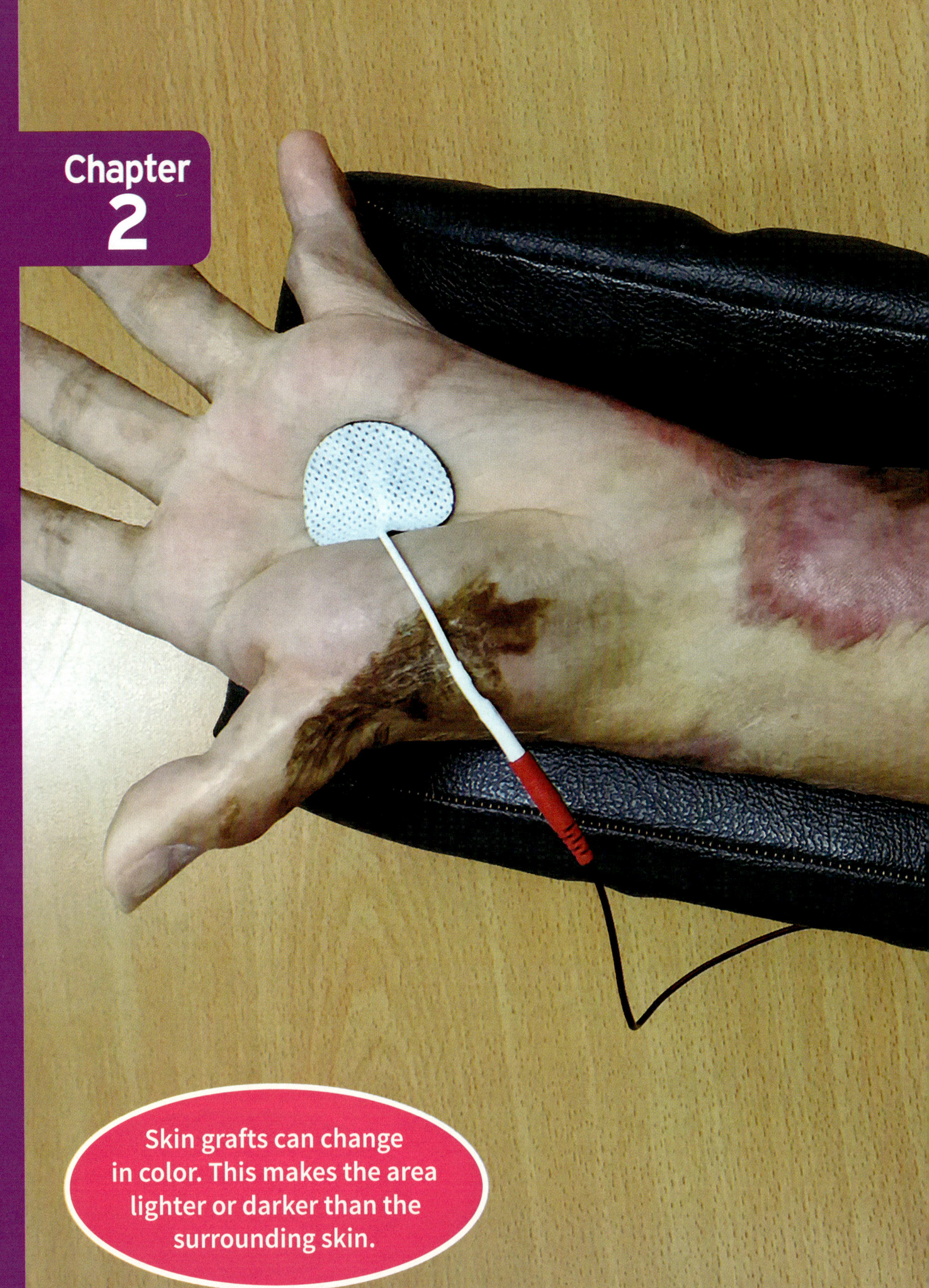

Skin grafts can change in color. This makes the area lighter or darker than the surrounding skin.

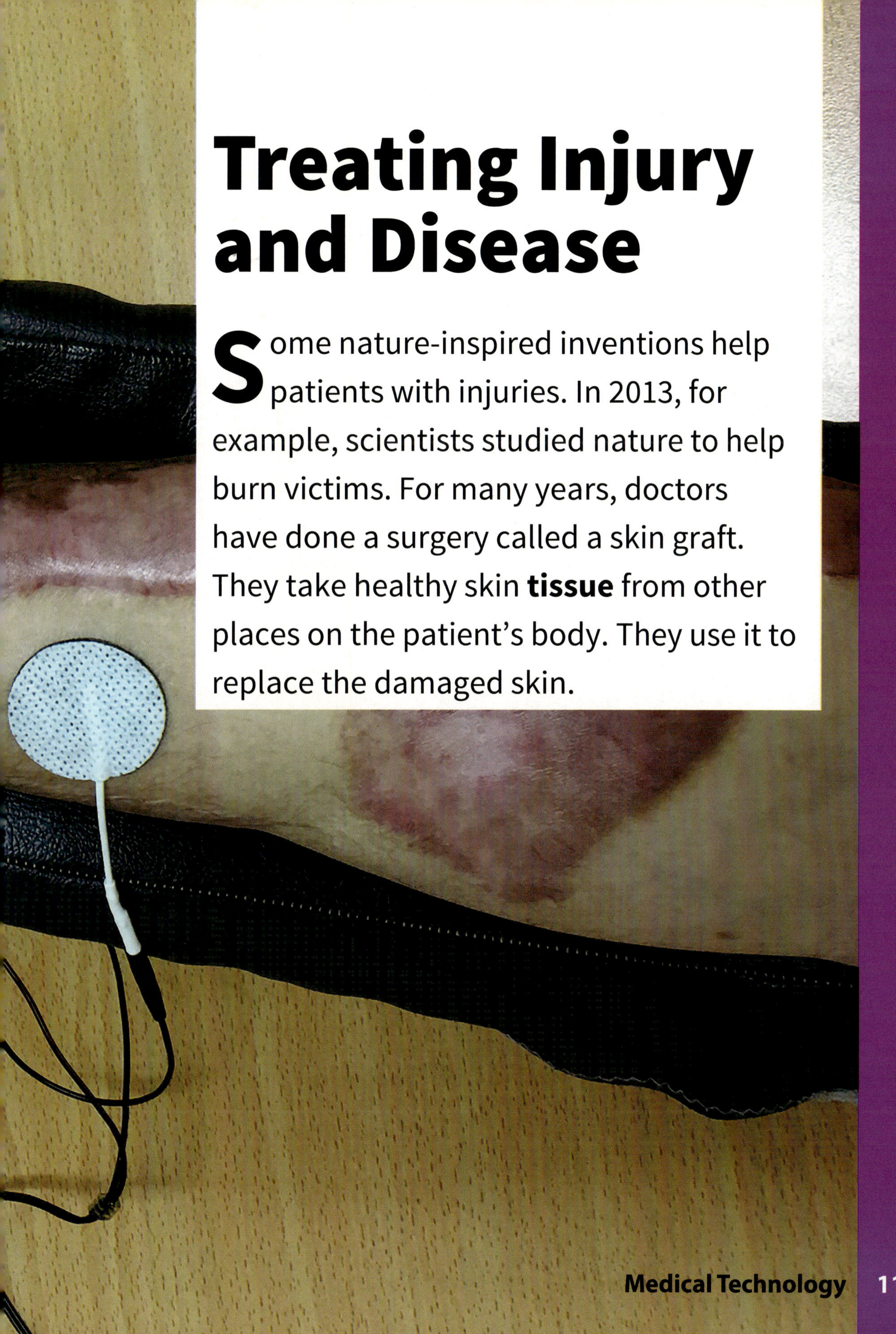

Treating Injury and Disease

Some nature-inspired inventions help patients with injuries. In 2013, for example, scientists studied nature to help burn victims. For many years, doctors have done a surgery called a skin graft. They take healthy skin **tissue** from other places on the patient's body. They use it to replace the damaged skin.

To improve skin grafts, scientists turned to flesh-grabbing worms. One type of worm uses its sharp spine to pierce its prey's flesh. Then it inflates its spiny head inside the tissue. This process helps the worm latch on.

There are more than 1,000 kinds of spiny headed worms.

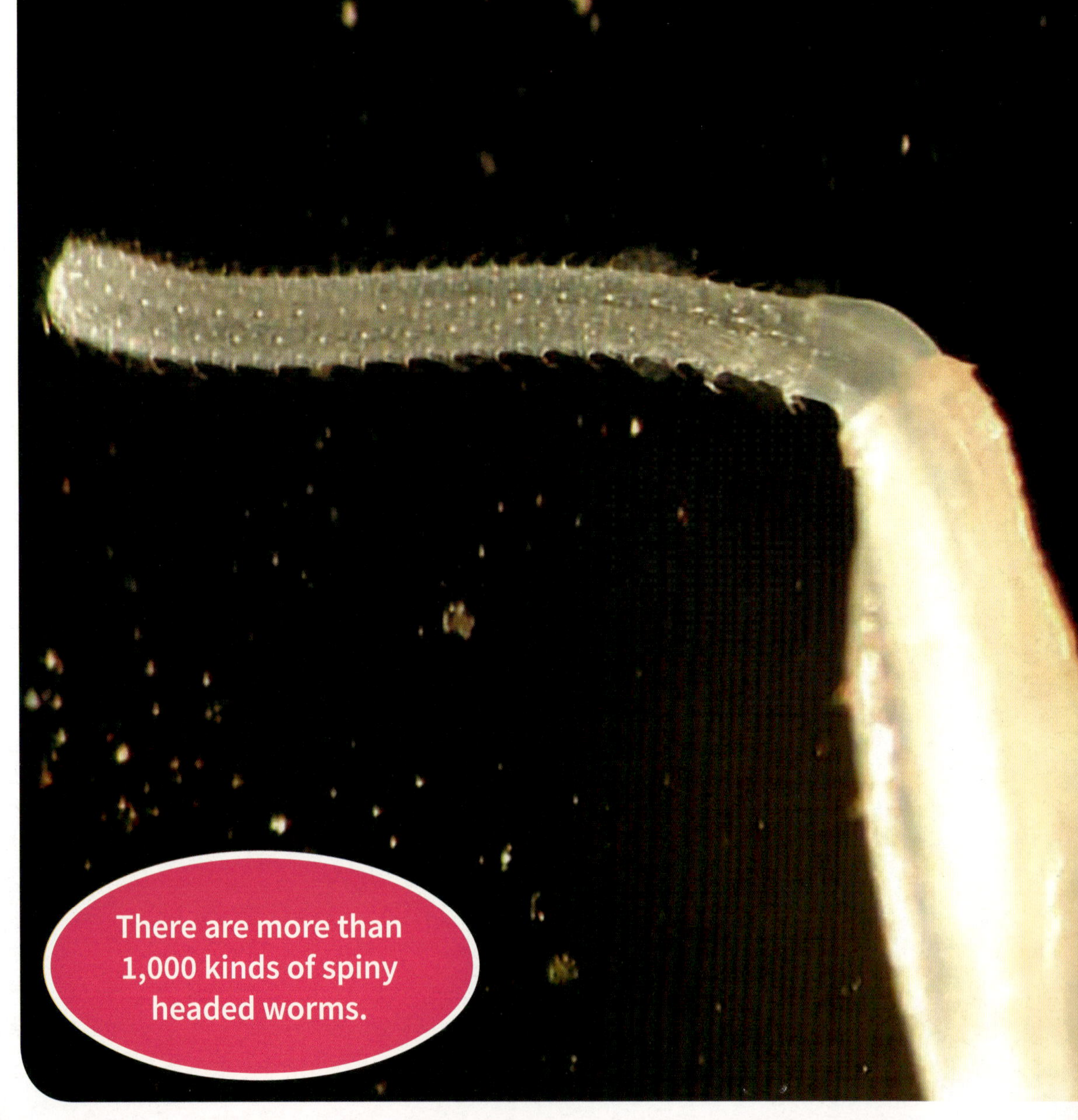

Scientists used the worm as a model for a new type of skin graft. In the improved process, doctors pierce burned skin with a patch of tiny needles. Similar to the worm's head, the tips of the needles inflate. They keep the healthy skin in place while the burned tissue heals.

Nature-inspired technology has also helped doctors treat certain diseases. One example is a **microchip** designed for cancer patients. Scientists based this idea on jellyfish. These sea creatures use their long tentacles to catch food. They can extend their tentacles far away from their bodies. This helps them grab food from a distance.

A Design for Many Uses

Doctors perform skin grafts for a variety of patients. Skin grafting can help treat skin infections and large wounds. It can also help treat skin cancer. This makes the worm-inspired skin graft all the more important. These skin grafts are three times stronger than other materials used in the past.

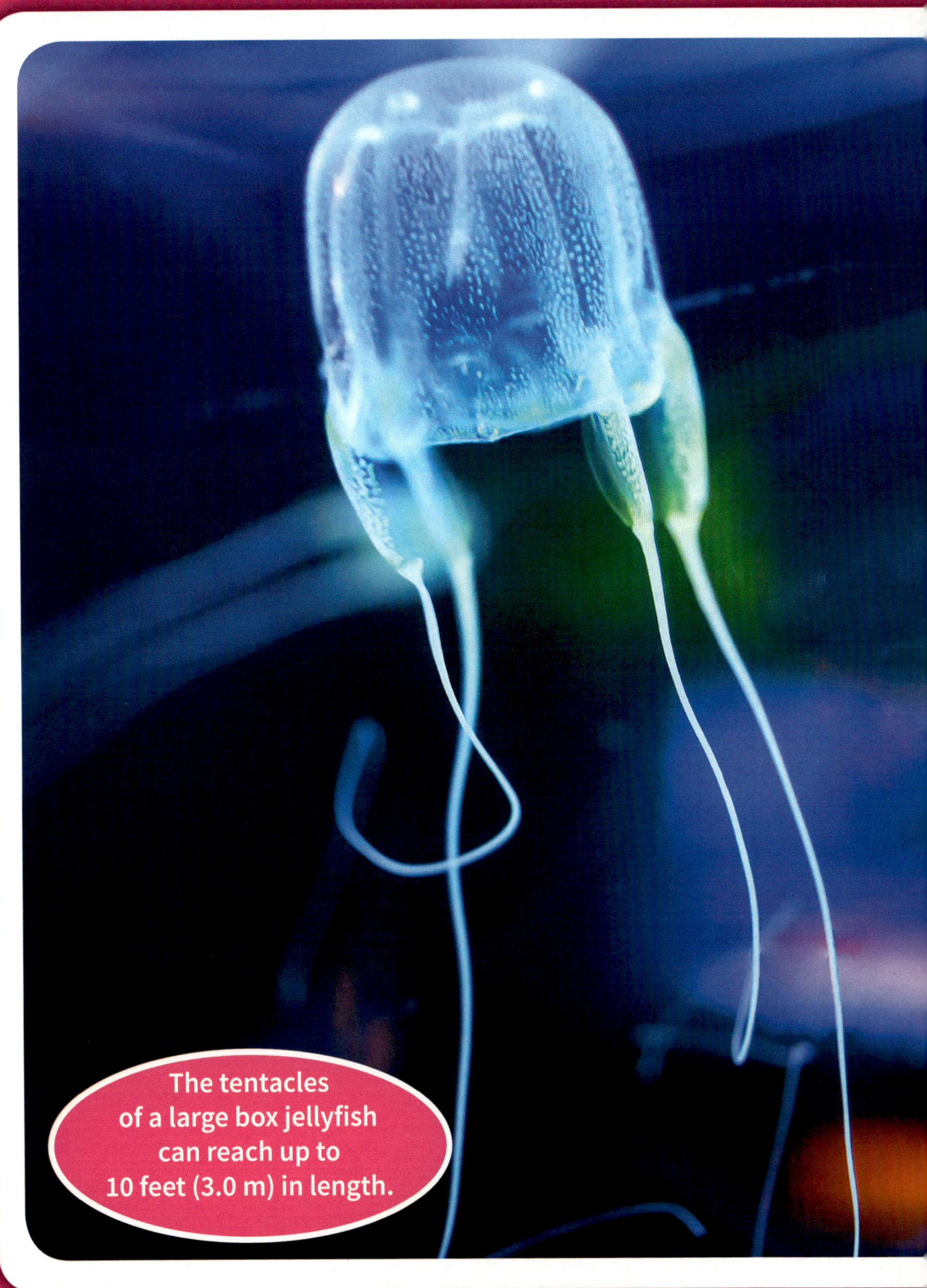

The tentacles of a large box jellyfish can reach up to 10 feet (3.0 m) in length.

In 2012, scientists created a microchip that would help them do something similar. The scientists combined strands of **DNA** to create a long, wispy material. One end of the material is attached to the microchip. The other end reaches into the patient's bloodstream. The strand grabs **cancer cells** and counts them. This cell count is very helpful to doctors. It lets them know whether or not the patient's medicine is working.

The new microchip can count cells 10 times faster than previous devices. This makes a great difference. Doctors can more quickly determine which medicines to use. They can also decide on the right amounts. As a result, patients are more likely to recover.

Chapter 3

Medicine made from the flower *Galanthus caucasicus* may improve patients' memory.

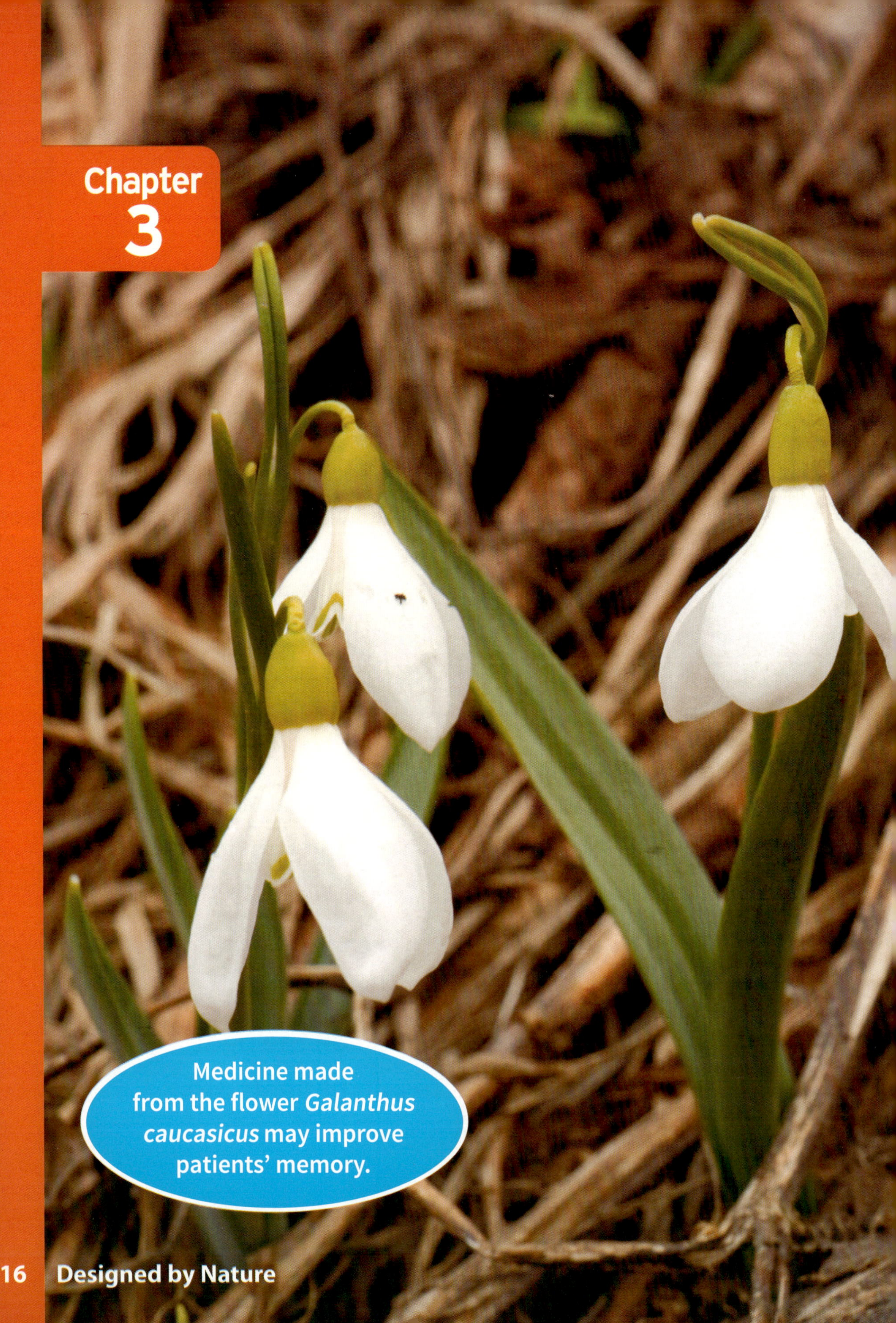

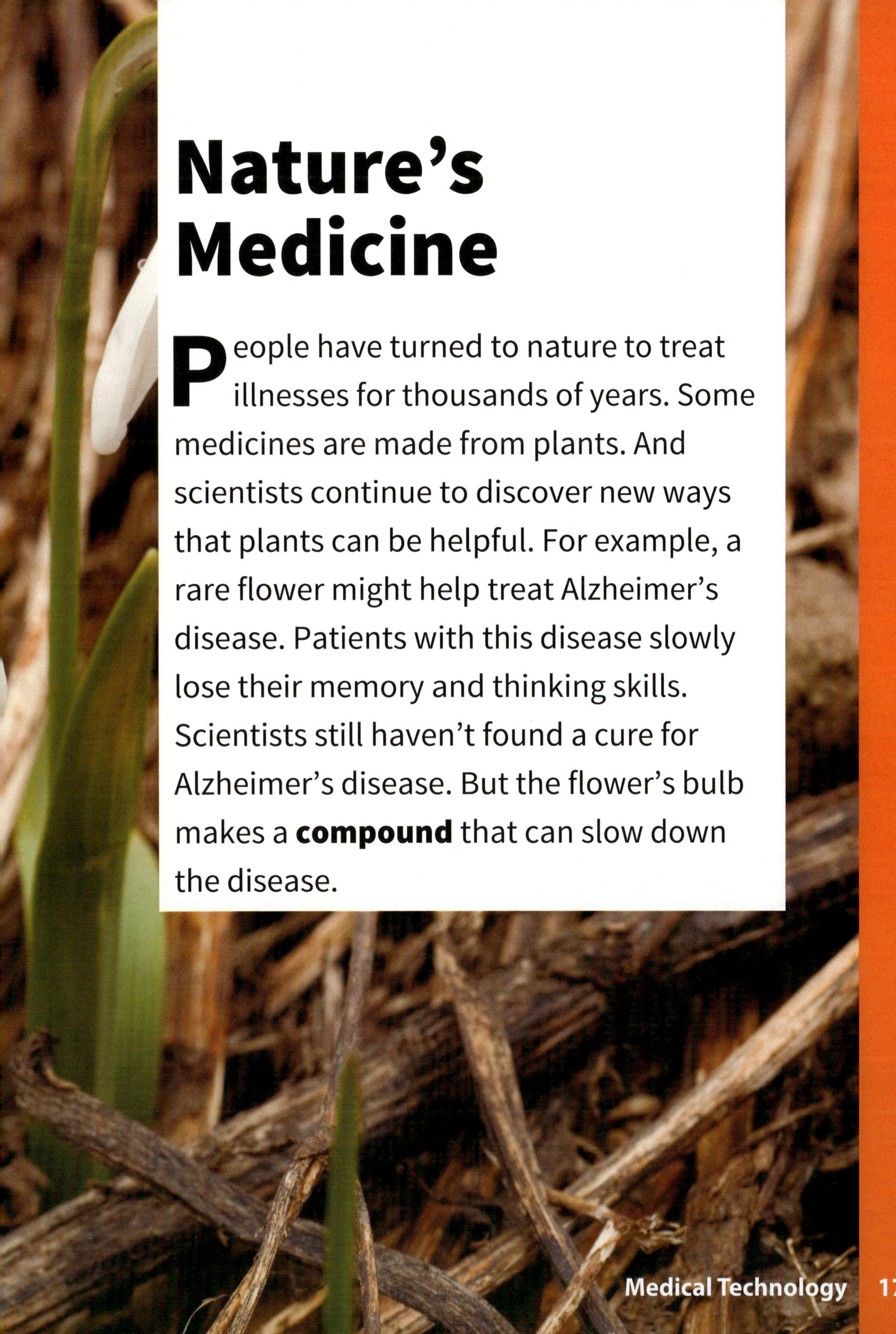

Nature's Medicine

People have turned to nature to treat illnesses for thousands of years. Some medicines are made from plants. And scientists continue to discover new ways that plants can be helpful. For example, a rare flower might help treat Alzheimer's disease. Patients with this disease slowly lose their memory and thinking skills. Scientists still haven't found a cure for Alzheimer's disease. But the flower's bulb makes a **compound** that can slow down the disease.

Using the flower as medicine would be expensive. It could also cause the flower to go **extinct**. So instead, scientists made a copy. To do so, they created a new chemical compound. It was similar to the flower's compound. And it had the same effect on the disease. This helped protect the rare flower. It also lowered the cost of making the medicine.

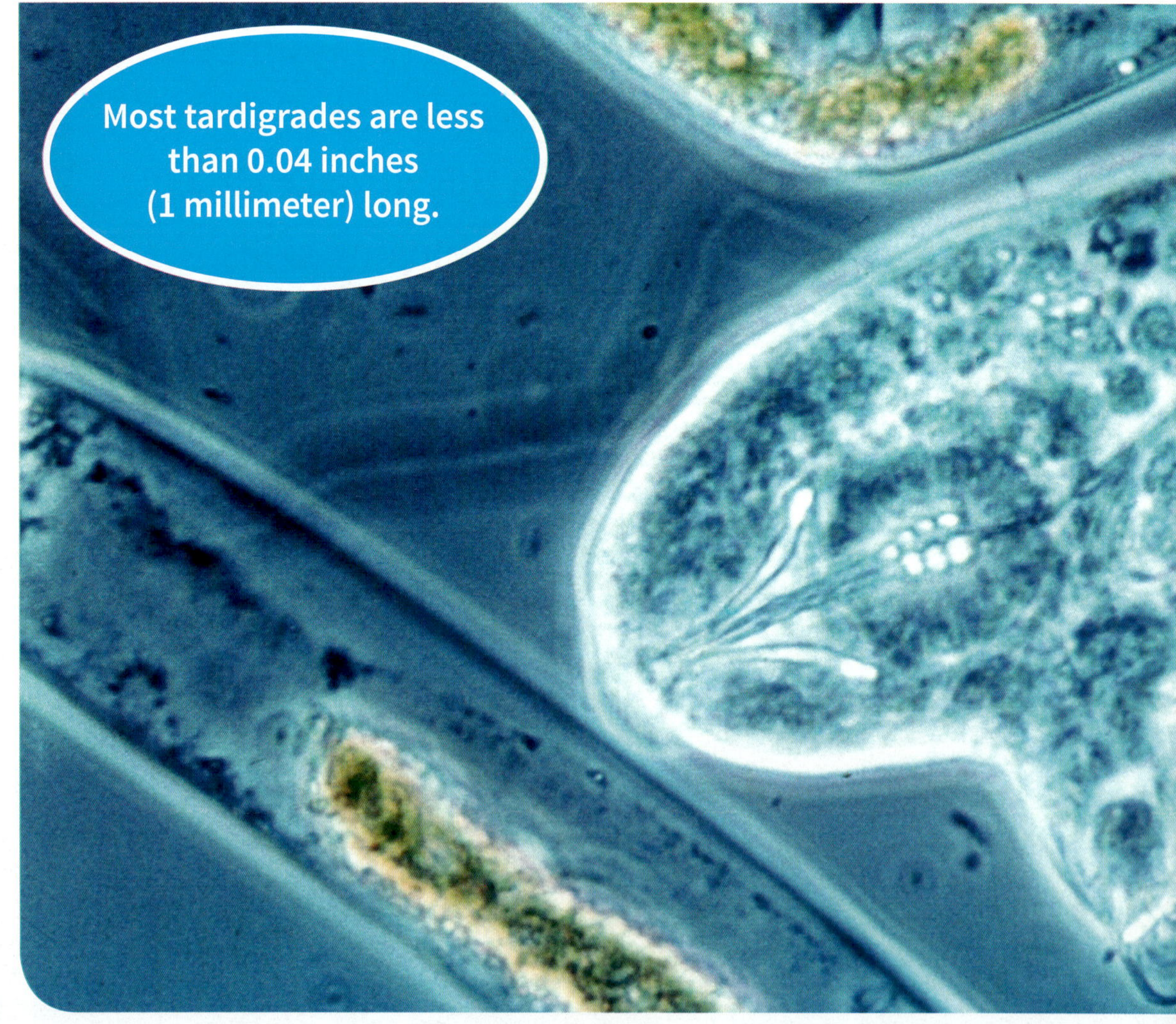

Scientists find ideas for medicine from animals, too. One example is a **vaccine** inspired by tardigrades. Tardigrades are eight-legged water animals. They're so small they can be seen only with a microscope. These tiny animals have amazing abilities. When tardigrades dry out, they become **dormant**. But water can make them active again. They can be revived even after 100 years.

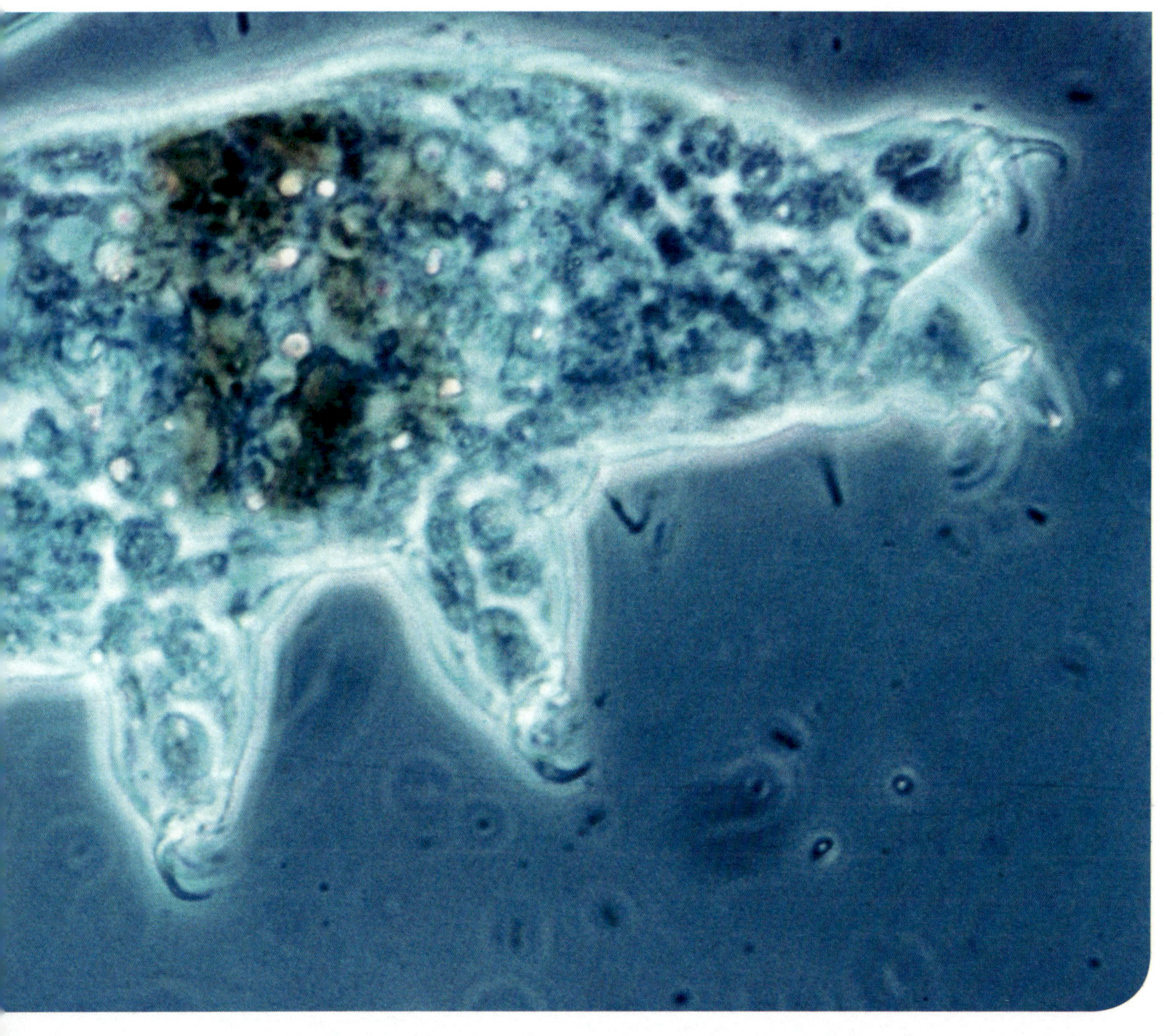

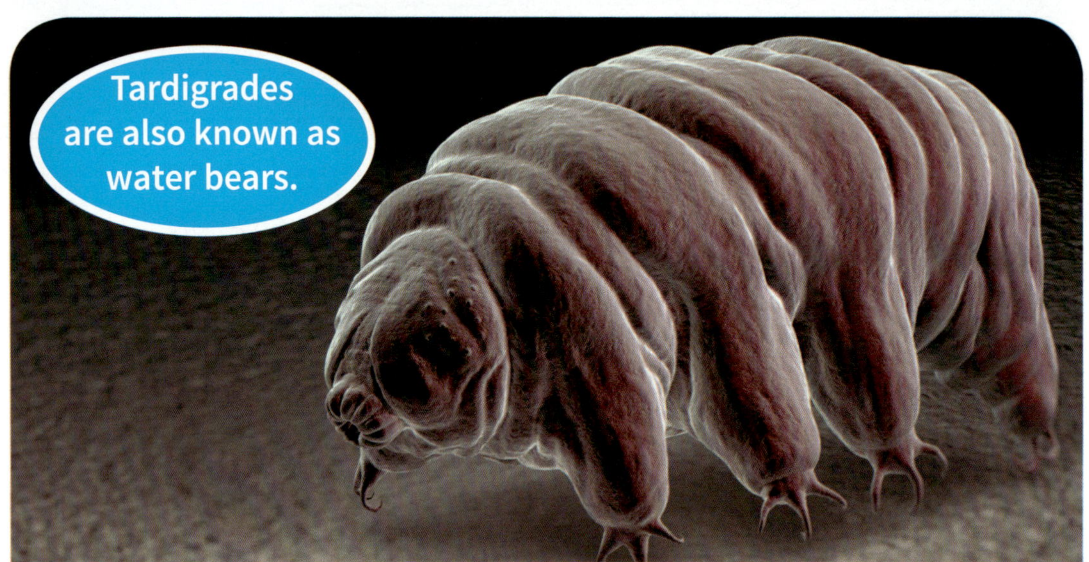

Tardigrades can also survive harsh conditions. They coat their cells with a type of sugar. The sugar protects the animal's cells. This helps them survive after being dried out for decades.

Treating High Blood Pressure

The jararaca is a snake found in South America. One bite from the snake can kill a human. The snake's venom causes the person's blood pressure to fall quickly. Scientists invented a chemical compound similar to the snake's venom. Now, doctors are using the compound to treat high blood pressure. Left untreated, high blood pressure can cause heart attacks. The snake-inspired medicine keeps blood pressure at a safe level.

Tardigrades inspired scientists to create a sugar-coated vaccine. Like other medicines, vaccines can **expire**. Most need to be kept in cold temperatures. The sugar coating helps the vaccine last longer. This way, the vaccine can be shipped across the world.

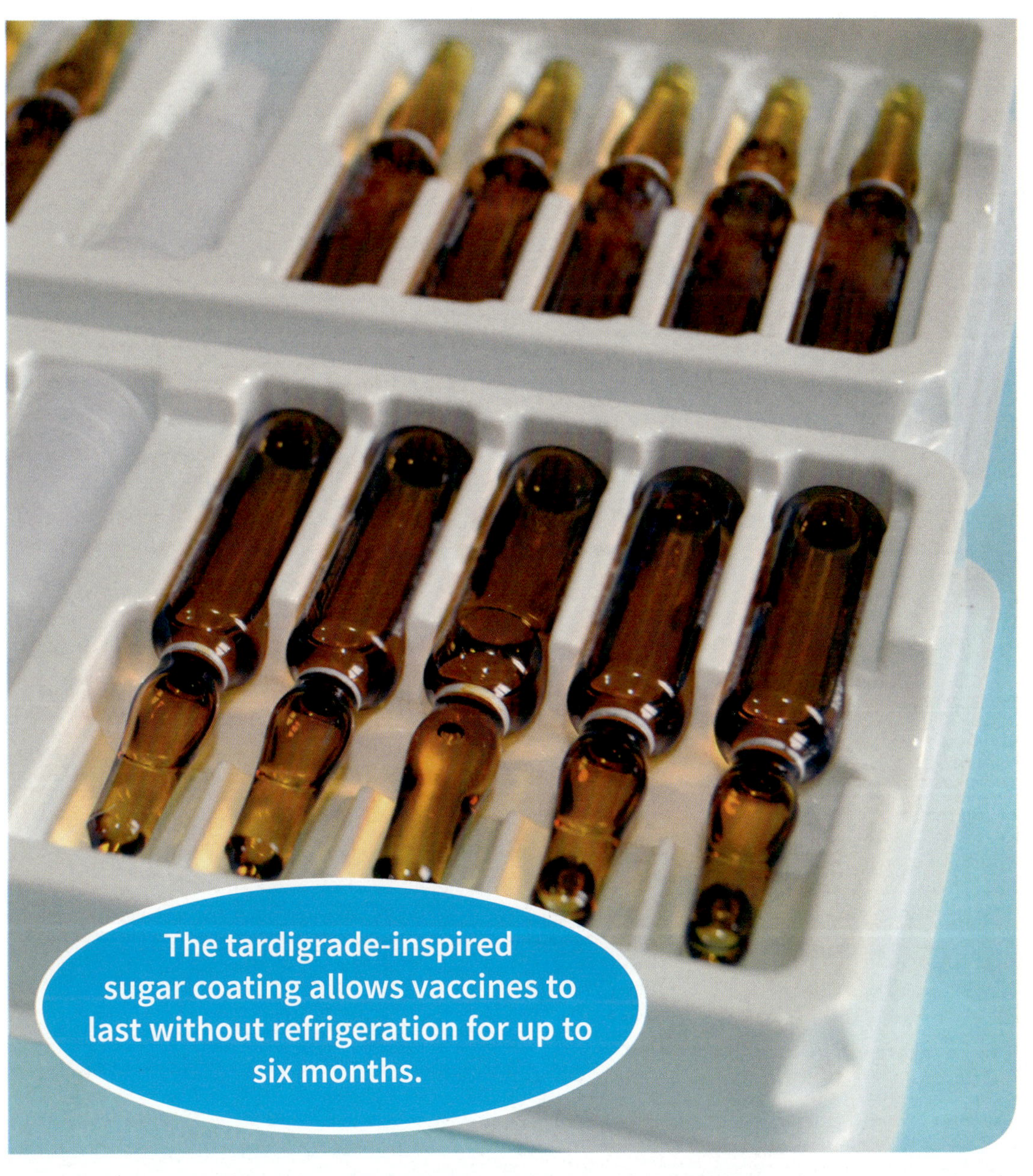

The tardigrade-inspired sugar coating allows vaccines to last without refrigeration for up to six months.

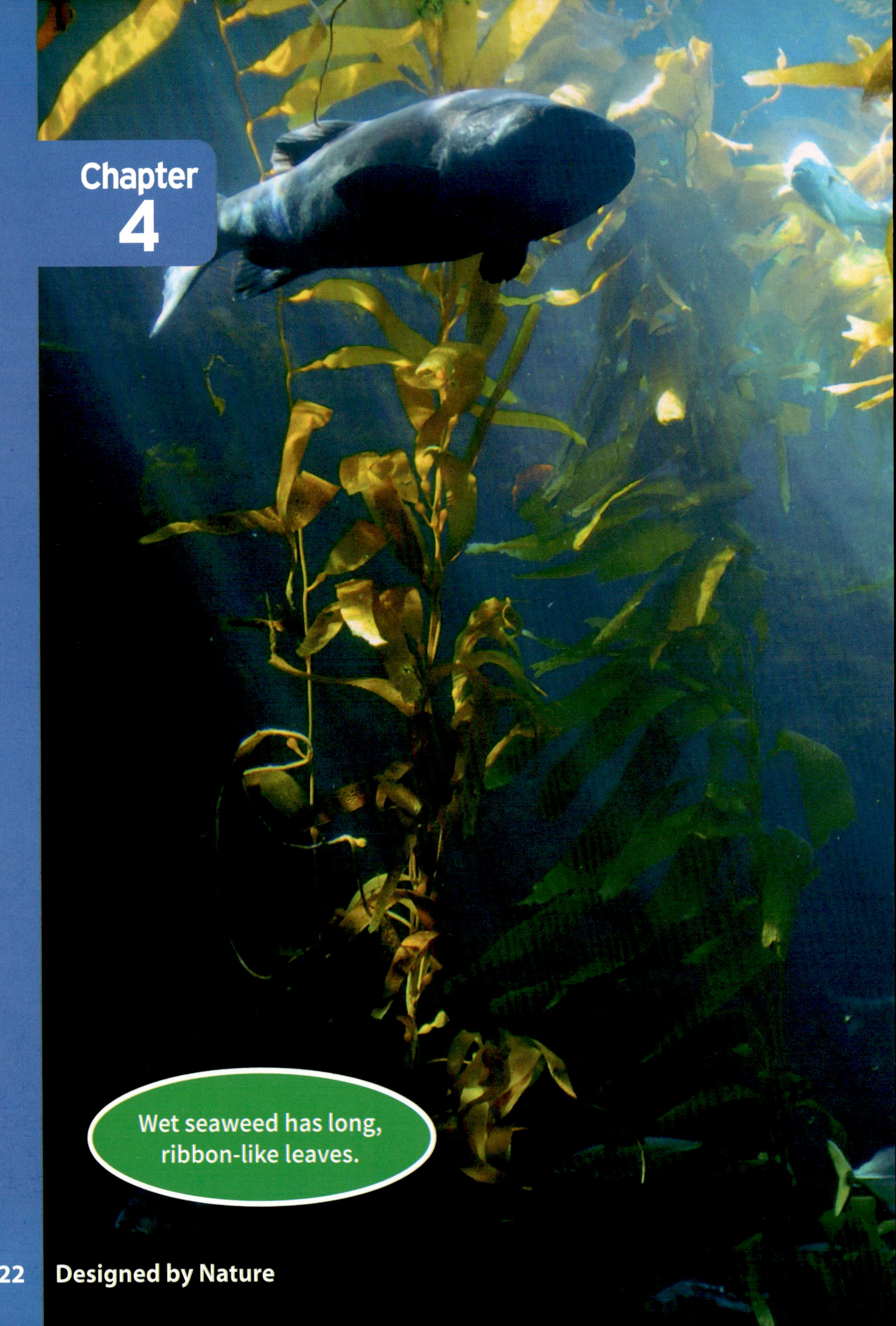

Chapter 4

Wet seaweed has long, ribbon-like leaves.

Future Inspiration

Inventing new medical technology takes years. The inventions must go through lots of testing. Scientists are working on many projects. One medical technology that is now in the works was inspired by seaweed. When seaweed is dry, it shrinks. But when it is wet, it expands.

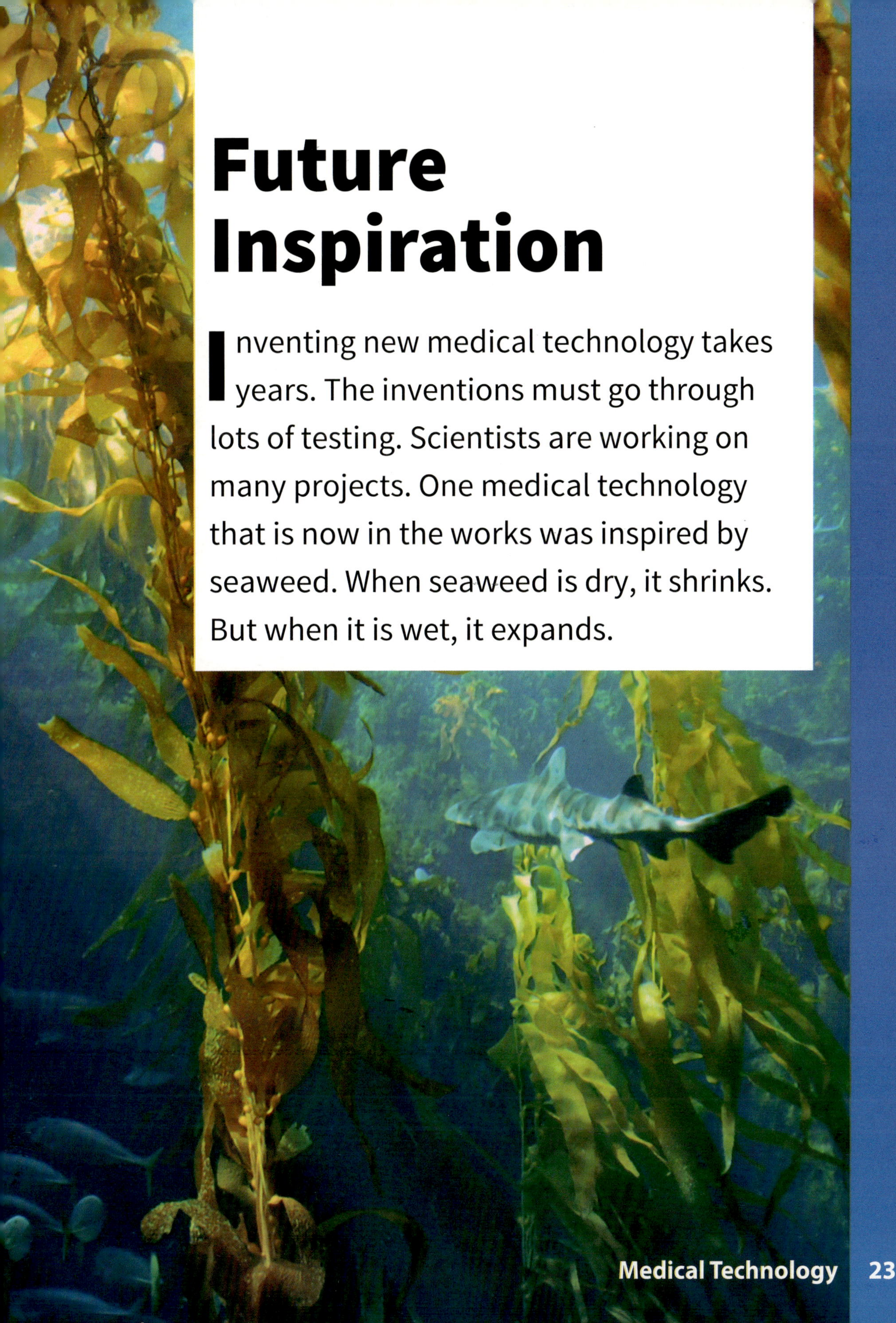

One North American porcupine quill has approximately **700 to 800 spikes** on its end.

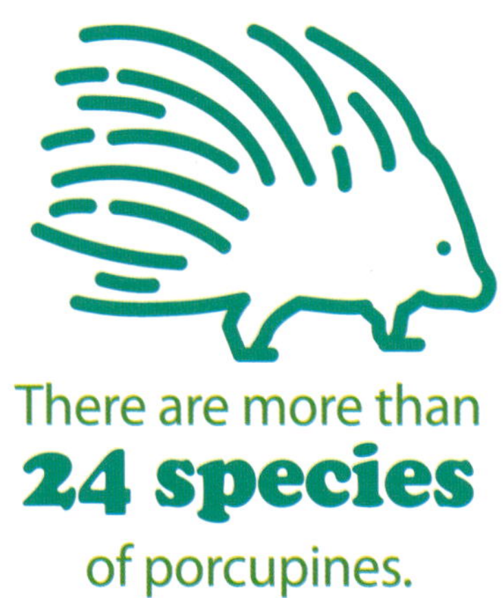

There are more than **24 species** of porcupines.

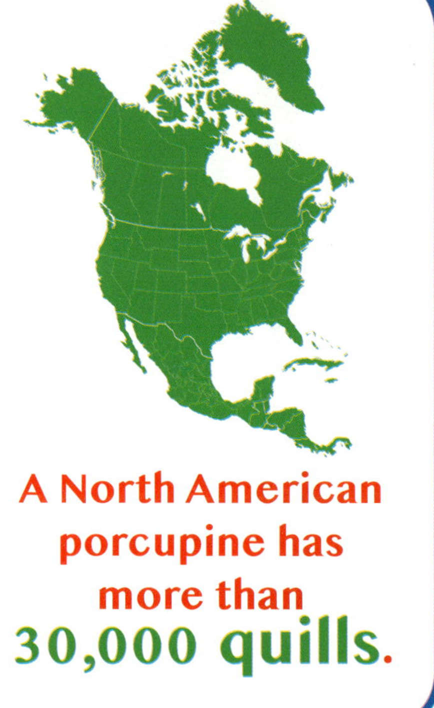

A North American porcupine has more than **30,000 quills.**

Scientists wanted to use the same method to send medicine into patients' bodies. The result was a new medical sponge. The sponge is made of a jelly that comes from seaweed.

First, doctors fill the sponge with medicine. Then they shrink the sponge so it is very small. They place the sponge inside a needle. This allows them to inject it into a part of the patient's body. Once there, the sponge expands. It slowly releases the medicine. Then it dissolves.

The sponge was first developed in 2012. However, it could be a while before doctors can use the tool. As of 2018, scientists were still testing it.

Scientists are also working on a new kind of staple. Doctors use staples to hold skin in place after surgery. Staples have two prongs that pierce the top layers of the skin. The new staples are based on porcupine quills. A porcupine quill has sharp spikes at its end. One scientist tested a quill by poking it into his skin. The quill made a small, clean hole. The spikes helped the quill go in easily.

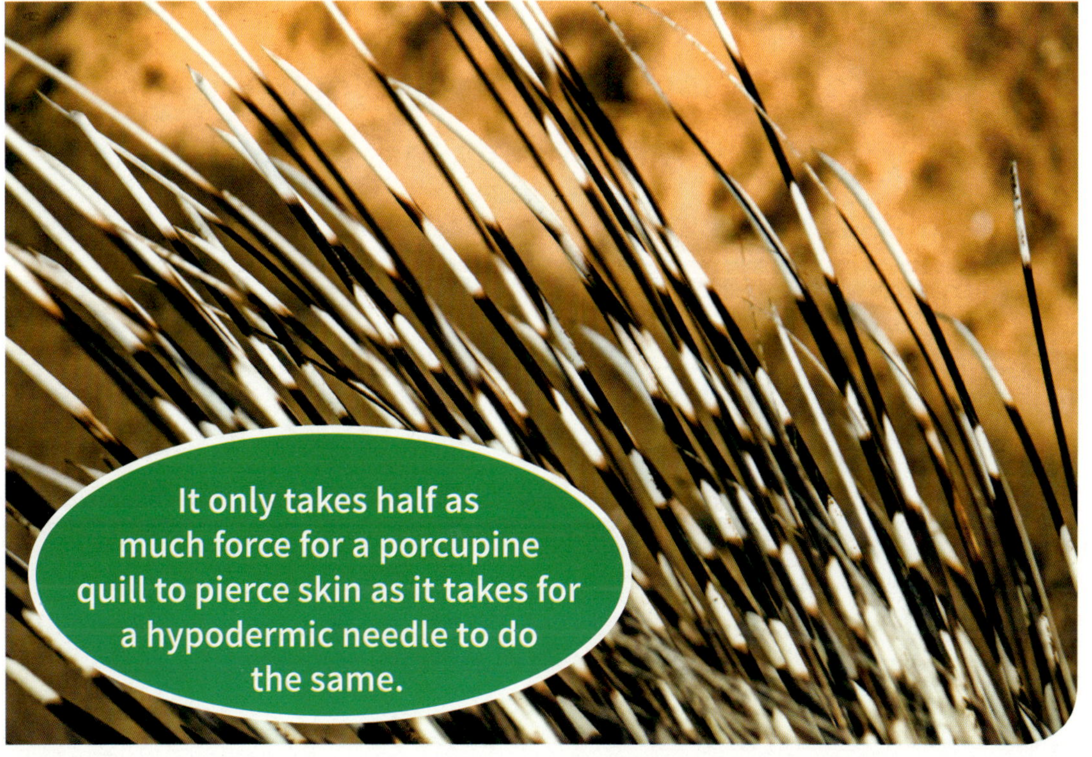

It only takes half as much force for a porcupine quill to pierce skin as it takes for a hypodermic needle to do the same.

Most surgical staples make large holes in the skin. This means more **bacteria** can enter the wound. The bacteria often cause infection. Similar to a quill, the new staples would have spikes. The spikes would allow the staple to make small holes. Infection would be less likely. The spikes would also keep the staple in place. Once the staple was no longer needed, it would dissolve inside the body. The staples are still being tested. But one day, they could help many patients in hospitals.

The world is full of fascinating animals and plants. As scientists study them, they continue to find new ideas for medical technology. Such technology does more than copy nature. It takes what works in nature and then builds upon it. In this way, the technology leaves a lasting mark on the future of medicine.

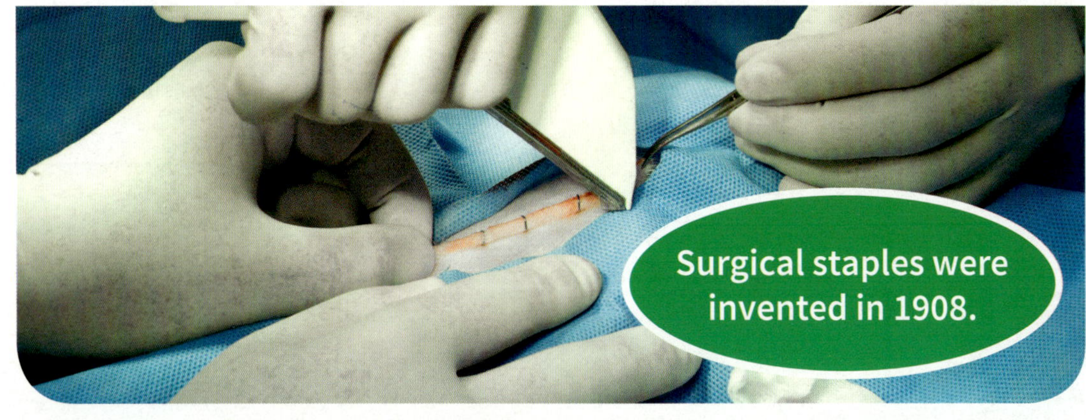

Surgical staples were invented in 1908.

Timeline

Humans have been using nature to develop medicine for many years. As people understand more about the natural world, they are able to make new kinds of medical tools and techniques.

2004 In the United States, the Food and Drug administration (FDA) declares that leeches used for therapy can be considered medical devices.

2008 New surgical tape, based on gecko skin, is invented as a tool to help replace sutures and staples.

2009 A biotech company in Florida develops a form of **artificial** shark skin. The pattern on the skin helps keep bacteria off its surface.

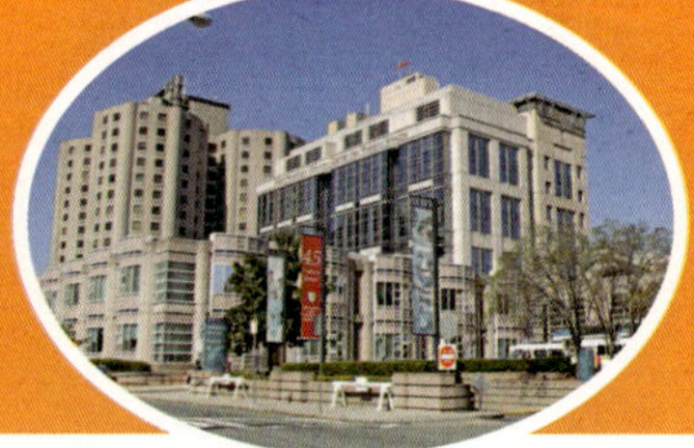

2013 Researchers at Boston's Brigham and Women's Hospital develop new microneedles based on the parasitic *Pomphorhynchus laevis* worms.

2014 University of Texas researchers develop a new kind of hypersensitive hearing aid based on the ears of parasitic flies.

2017 Researchers examine the blood of animals such as Komodo dragons to determine if they have antibacterial properties that can be copied for medicine.

Medical Inventions Map

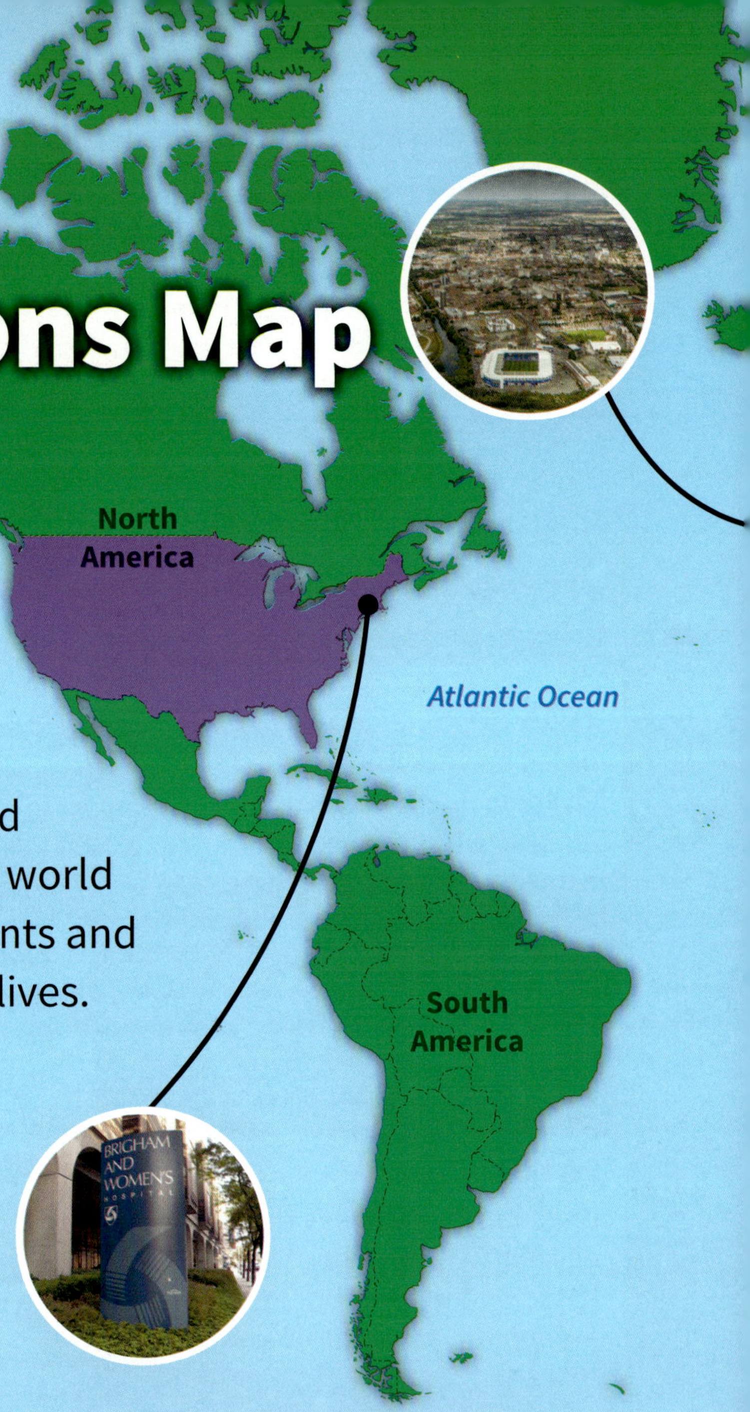

Pacific Ocean

North America

Atlantic Ocean

South America

People have used nature to treat injuries for thousands of years. Today, laboratories and companies around the world are examining how plants and animals can help save lives.

Legend
Water
Land
N W E S
Scale
0
2,000 Miles
2,000 Kilometers

BRIGHAM AND WOMEN'S HOSPITAL

United States
Bioengineer Jeffrey Karp was inspired by gecko feet to make surgical tape while working at Brigham and Women's Hospital (BWH) in Boston, Massachusetts.

Great Britain
Nova Laboratories, in Leicester, Great Britain, is one of several companies inspired by tardigrades to research ways to preserve vaccines.

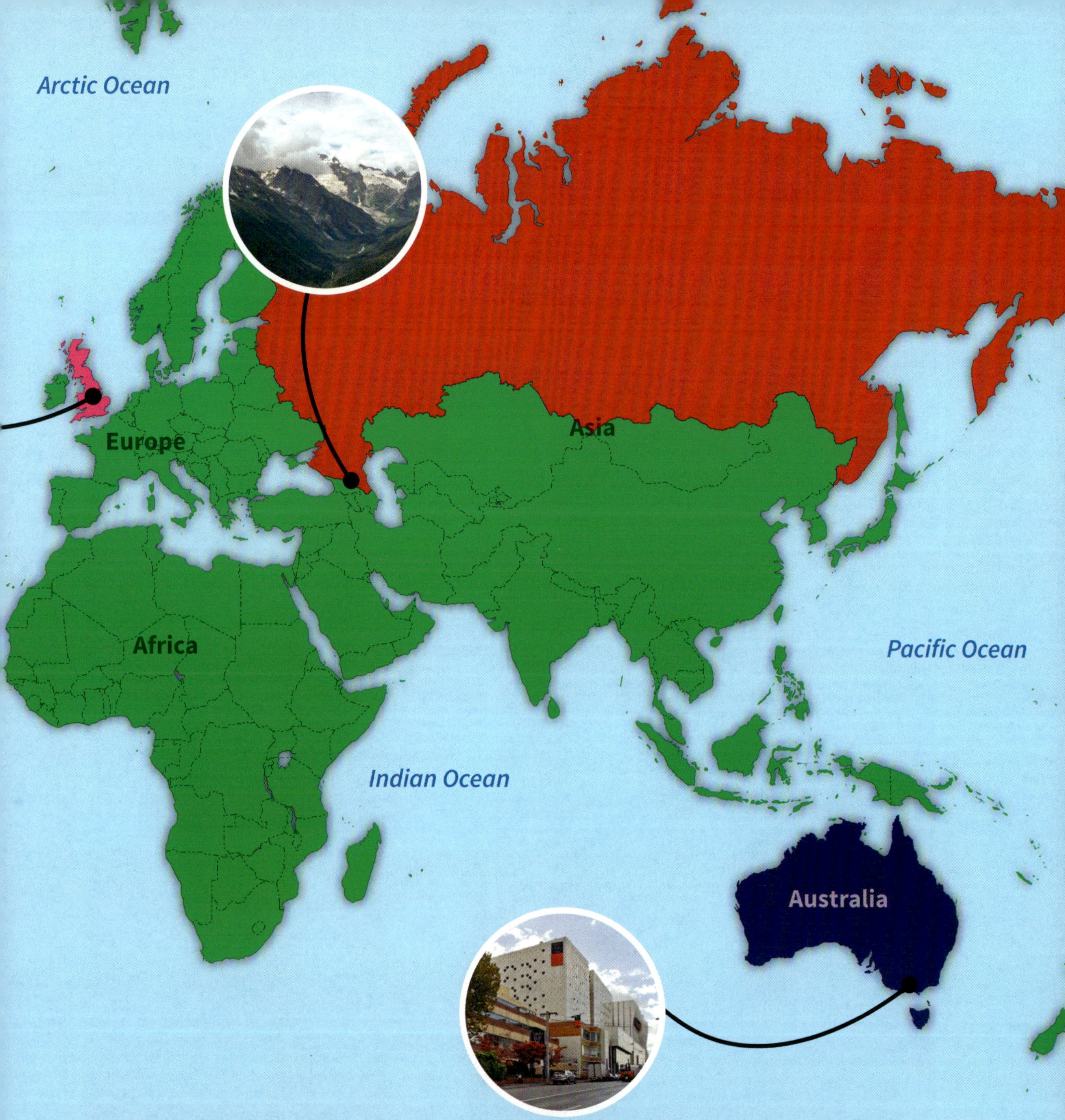

Russia

In the 1950s, people in Russia's Caucasus Mountains used snowdrop flowers to help with head pains. Today, chemicals from the plants may help fight Alzheimer's.

Australia

In 2013, a study headed by Professor Elena Ivanova of Australia's Swinburne University of Technology studied how the structure of a clanger cicada's body kills bacteria. This structure could be used to coat surfaces and help control disease.

Quiz

1 How many spikes are on the end of a North American porcupine quill?

Answer: 700 to 800

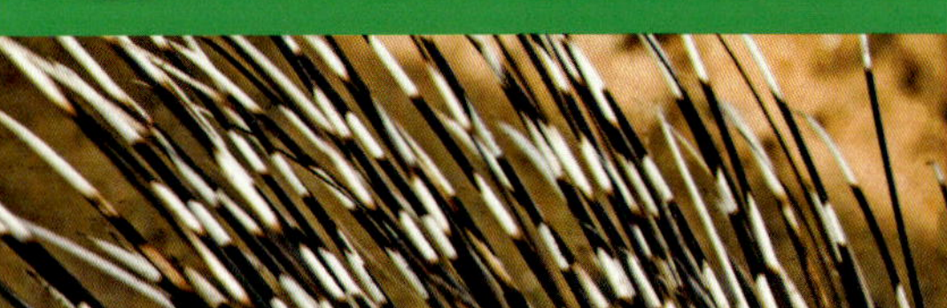

2 Which bioengineer developed surgical tape based on gecko feet?

Answer: Jeffrey Karp

3 What is another name for a tardigrade?

Answer: A water bear

4 How many hospitals in France tested sandcastle-worm-based glue in 2016?

Answer: Four

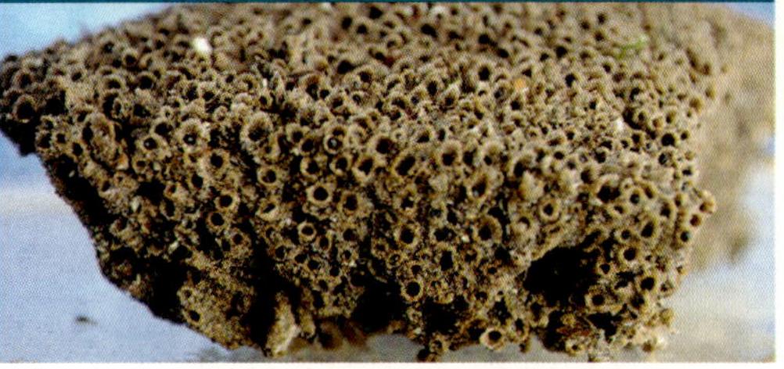

5 When was the first surgical tape invented?

Answer: 1845

6 What do the tips of worm-based skin graft needles do?

Answer: Inflate

7 What animals were declared to be medical devices by the FDA in 2004?

Answer: Leeches

8 What happens to a tardigrade when it dries out?

Answer: It becomes dormant

9 What animals inspired scientists to make a type of microchip in 2012?

Answer: Jellyfish

10 How many species of gecko are there?

Answer: More than 1,000

Key Words

artificial: made by humans instead of occurring naturally

bacteria: single-celled living things. They can be useful or harmful.

cancer cells: abnormal cells that divide and grow in the body

compound: a substance that is made by combining two or more chemical elements

DNA: the genetic material in the cells of living organisms

dormant: alive but not active, as if in a deep sleep

expire: to reach the end of the time when something is useful

extinct: no longer living on Earth

microchip: a small piece of hardware that has tiny electrical circuits

tissue: a group of similar cells that have a certain job or function

vaccine: a substance that prevents a person from getting a disease

Index

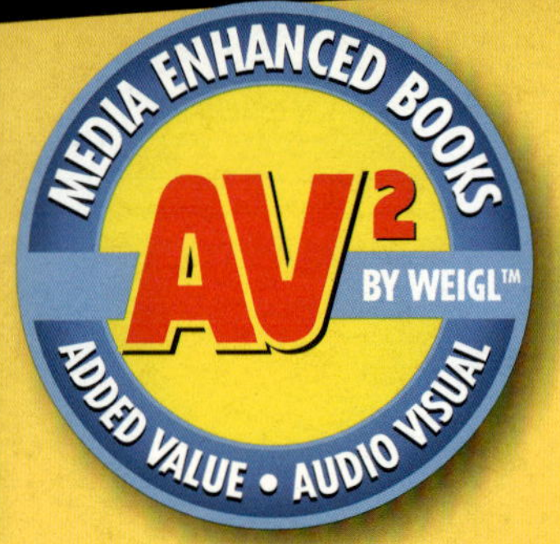

Log on to www.av2books.com

AV² by Weigl brings you media enhanced books that support active learning. Go to www.av2books.com, and enter the special code found on page 2 of this book. You will gain access to enriched and enhanced content that supplements and complements this book. Content includes video, audio, weblinks, quizzes, a slide show, and activities.

AV² Online Navigation

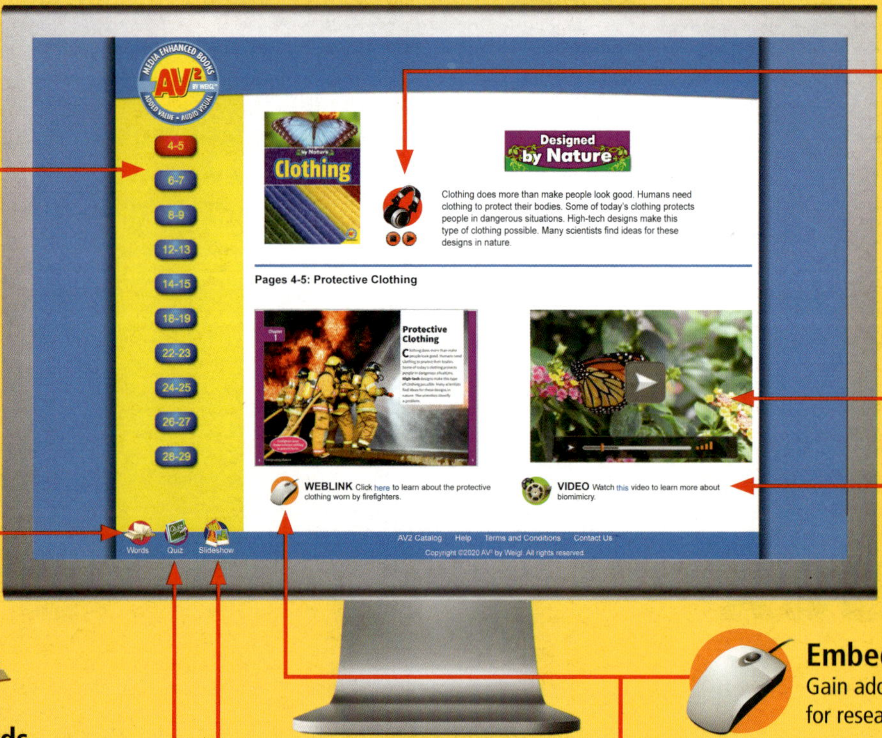

Audio
Listen to sections of the book read aloud.

Book Pages
AV² pages directly correspond to pages in the book.

Video
Watch informative video clips.

Embedded Weblinks
Gain additional information for research.

Key Words
Study vocabulary, and complete a matching word activity.

Try This!
Complete activities and hands-on experiments.

Quizzes
Test your knowledge.

Slide Show
View images and captions, and prepare a presentation.

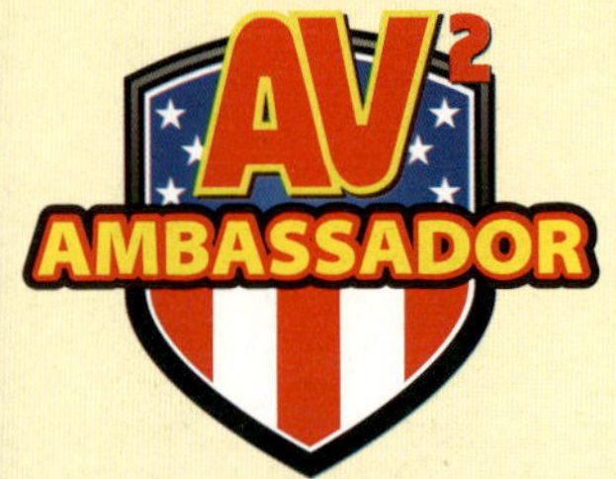

AV² was built to bridge the gap between print and digital. We encourage you to tell us what you like and what you want to see in the future.

Sign up to be an AV² Ambassador at www.av2books.com/ambassador.

Due to the dynamic nature of the Internet, some of the URLs and activities provided as part of AV² by Weigl may have changed or ceased to exist. AV² by Weigl accepts no responsibility for any such changes. All media enhanced books are regularly monitored to update addresses and sites in a timely manner. Contact AV² by Weigl at 1-866-649-3445 or av2books@weigl.com with any questions, comments, or feedback.